RESTARTING
THE WORLD

RESTARTING THE WORLD

A NEW NORMAL AFTER A PANDEMIC

H. Dorman Wright

Bryn Edwards

H. NORMAN WRIGHT
AND BRYN EDWARDS

B&H
PUBLISHING
NASHVILLE, TENNESSEE

Published by B&H Publishing Group
Nashville, Tennessee

Dewey Decimal Classification: 158
Subject Heading: EMOTIONS / COVID-
19—(DISEASE) / LIFE SKILS

Cover design by B&H Publishing Group. Cover
photo by fotoeventis/Getty Images.

Contents

CHAPTER 1

The World Stood Still

No one knew what was about to take place. The year 2020 began like any other year—with New Year's resolutions and hopes and dreams abounding from coast to coast. Yet 2020 held more unpleasant surprises than anyone could have imagined.

We hear about events throughout the nation with real-time communication and media coverage, and we have seen many tragedies and storms unfold across our country in the past few years. In California it's the yearly firestorms or the threat of the "Big One" that could happen at any moment. More than thirty years ago, I experienced an earthquake while playing racquetball with a friend. At first, I thought the aerobics class on the floor above was louder than usual, but realized it was more when the walls began to sway back and forth. When the lights went out, my friend and I ran for the door and grasped to find the recessed door handle, shattering a few fingernails in our haste. Hearts pounding, we ran outside as the ground continued to shake. We later learned we were seven miles from the epicenter of the 5.9 quake that caused several fires, injured many people, and caused eight deaths.

Hurricanes flood the Gulf and East Coast causing millions of dollars' worth of damage, and the Midwest experiences devastating tornadoes. And tornadoes are not always limited to the Midwest. Several years ago, we experienced a full-sized twister on our street in southern California. My wife, Joyce, was working in the yard and felt some strange and strong winds. Realizing something was wrong, she went inside and shut the door. The winds continued, and it seemed as if the air was being sucked out of the house. Not knowing what was happening, she shut herself in an inside room. About this time a neighbor turned the corner on her way home just in time to see the twister set down in the middle of the block and come toward her. She drove her car into the garage and ran into the house before the tornado ripped the large trees from her front yard.

Mass shootings happen all too often and tragically disrupt communities taking the lives of the innocent. I've ministered to victims and communities after these tragedies have taken place throughout the country, and I spent more than a year helping twenty-one students and staff members deal with the trauma at a local high school where a student was shot and wounded by another student. These events break our hearts and each time we lose a little more of our sense of security, but the vast majority of our population is not personally affected.

Who would have imagined that several individuals gathering at an airport on a Sunday morning to travel to a girl's youth basketball tournament would never reach their destination? When we heard the story, time seemed to slow down. On January 26, 2020, we lost a legend—a basketball player known for his God-given ability, drive, competitiveness, and generousness. He was an icon to a generation of athletes and a pillar in the sports world, due to his twenty-year career on the Los Angeles Lakers. Kobe Bryant was not alone in the helicopter crash that killed eight other people besides himself. I ministered to some of those who were directly affected by this tragic loss—relatives, classmates, teachers, and friends. The ripple effects impacted the family members and friends of each person who died that day. As a country we collectively grieved this tragedy, not realizing there was an unforeseen event on the horizon that would affect us as a nation in ways we had not experienced in our lifetime. This was a new type of storm. It was quiet. It was subtle. It crept in without our knowing its presence.

It started as a rumbling. We were learning about the Coronavirus in bits and pieces as it infected many people in China and started making its way through Europe. Little did we know the entire country would soon be shutting down, and for much longer than anyone suspected. Schools throughout the country sent students home with plans for them to return to school a few weeks later. Restrictions on gathering affected every area of our lives. Many businesses shut their doors, and employees were sent home not knowing when they would be returning to work.

Daily the news changed. It was recommended that anyone over the age of sixty-five "shelter in place" and avoid public places. The term *defiant elderly* was given to the senior citizens who chose not to stay at home and continued to go about their daily business. Before we knew it, a *quarantine* with no specific end in sight was put in place for the residents in many states, and we were told to only leave the house when necessary. Life as we knew it completely changed. The pandemic had landed in America, and the news we were hearing was not good. New York, especially New York City, was seeing high numbers of people diagnosed with COVID-19 daily—and this was expected to hit the rest of the states in the same manner. We asked ourselves questions, wondering how this would affect our families. *Will I get COVID-19? Will I die? Will someone in my family die? When will life return to normal? When will I return to work?*

Where were you when the world stopped? There is no other way to describe the numb feeling. We vacillate from belief to unbelief, from acceptance to denial, wondering what went wrong and what the future will hold. And at times it feels like the earth is standing still. With the shelter-in-place order, the busyness of our daily lives came to a halt.

There was another day that felt like the earth stood still—September 11, 2001. We watched our televisions as the tragic events unfolded. In October, I went to New York to minister to those who had experienced firsthand the destruction that was left from the falling towers. It seems like it was just yesterday, and the current events bring it back to mind because of the devastation COVID-19 has caused. But I also remember a night in November 2001—the TV was on, but this time the news wasn't replaying the collapsing towers; this time country singer Alan Jackson was debuting his new song "Where Were You (When the World Stopped Turning)." The words touched me emotionally since I knew personally how lives had been changed. And as the nation healed from an uncontrollable event, we prayed this wouldn't happen again.

Most of us believe that we are in control of our lives—that is, until a tragedy strikes. We learned that in September 2001, and we learned it again in March 2020. The control we thought we had was taken from us along with our sense of well-being. The loss of control affects us in many ways: fear, anxiety, frustration, insecurity, anger, loss, and loneliness (created by the stay-at-home orders and social distancing). But there is a flip side to losing control—learning to be content in all circumstances, trusting completely that God is in control, and sharing this hope with others.

The United States spent more than an entire year watching the ebb and flow of COVID-19 as the number of infections and deaths rose and fell intermittently. We don't know what the future will hold. As we immerge from the isolation, life will be different. We wonder if it's over or if it will rear its ugly head again; will it disappear completely or be followed by an even worse pandemic in the future? As you read through this book, let's look at both the good and the bad, finding new ways to cope with uncertainty and loss of control.

Even in the midst of chaos, we can still find hope and find peace. "Now may the God of hope fill you with all joy and peace as you believe so that you may overflow with hope by the power of the Holy Spirit" (Rom. 15:13).

CHAPTER 2

Perpetual White Water

Our lives were disrupted—there is no doubt about it. And no one was immune. Daily routines we took for granted ended as quarantining dragged on for months. We were cut off from others and our emotions ran amuck. Some whose lives had been dictated by busyness found thankfulness, peace, and a sense of family unity. For others, depression, anger, and loneliness set in quickly. Some lost their sense of purpose being left alone with their thoughts. Many of us found ourselves floating somewhere in between "I can do this" and "When will this end?"

What is it like to have your life turned upside down?

You may have experienced this kind of upheaval before. Sudden change has the power to create chaos in your life. But did you also experience positive changes? Were you able to make the best of things? Did you hover between loss and gain? This has been a difficult journey.

As you read the descriptive terms below, circle the side you relate to at this time or put an X in the middle if you bounce between one and the other. We all have preconceived ideas of what we think we are experiencing, but most discover a number of surprises.

Hopeful	Hopeless
Fearful	Fearless
Loss	Gain
Sadness	Joy
Peace	Conflict
Depression	Vitality
Connect	Disconnect
Energetic	Drained
Purposeful	Purposeless
Renewed	Stuck

As you read through these words again, stop and think about how your life has changed since March 2020. How have you responded? Change is at the core of our lives. We may try to avoid it, but like a giant octopus its arms have encircled us, bringing our lives to a halt.

We have two choices. We can learn to accept and use the changes, or we can let them dominate our lives.

> Resisting change wears down our bodies, taxes our minds, and deflates our spirits. We keep doing the things that have always worked before with depressingly diminishing results. We expend precious energy looking around for someone to blame—ourselves, another person, or the world. We worry obsessively. We get stuck in the past, lost in bitterness or anger. Or we fall into denial—*everything's fine, I don't have to do anything differently.* Or magical thinking—*something or someone will come along to rescue me from having to change.* We don't want to leave the cozy comfort of the known and familiar for the scary wilderness of that which we've never experienced. And so, we rail against it and stay stuck.[1]

The former publisher of a major newspaper said this about the crash in 2007: "Anybody who professes to be able to tell you what things will be like in ten years is on some kind of drug." Once again this is true—the big picture is always changing, and our future is unknown. We don't have a clue about what our lives will be like in six months, one year, five years. The only thing any of us know for certain is that life changed at a rapid pace in 2020 and it will continue to change. Organizational consultant Peter Vails refers to this time of turbulence and uncertainty as "permanent white water." We can't see exactly where the submerged rocks are, but when we're tossed out of the boat, we want to make sure we know how to swim, not sink. Even experienced rafters know they're going to be thrown in the water at some point. The difference between them and the rest of us is that they're prepared to get bounced out and to recover swiftly. They expect the white water. And so should we as we find ourselves in uncharted waters.[2]

Where are you? Are you using change for your own growth or do you feel smothered by uncertainty? Are you allowing it to dominate your life? We all have a choice. Change gives us the opportunity to adapt and allow the change to refine us. It can be uncomfortable, but it's how we survive.

One of the advantages of what's happening right now is that it's happening to everyone. Whether you're coping with what to do with your kids while you're working at home, attending church in person or continuing to watch online, or whether or not to wear a mask as the mandates lift, you're not alone. Don't worry about what anyone else thinks—they're busy making their own decisions as they venture back into the world. Remembering we're all in a similar boat can be helpful.

Focusing on the upside of adapting is one of the best things we can do. Psychologists call this reframing.[3]

If you wonder what's going on with your life, it's normal. It might be new, it might be intense, but it's normal.

The brain is an internal problem-solving survival mechanism. It's beautiful. (Be sure to read *How to Keep Your Brain Young* by H. Norman Wright.) When there is a clear and present danger, our brains unleash a cascade of hormones meant to help us quickly escape. The nervous system shifts into high alert. The healthy, well-functioning brain helps us either escape the danger or fight off whatever has threatened our safety. Once the danger has passed, the body is meant to return to its calm, non-anxious, low-stress state. We push ourselves into exhaustion, trying to keep ourselves safe.[4]

As I said earlier, there are two ways to respond to change you didn't ask for: deny it or accept it. We get to choose to take positive steps to get the most out of change, or we choose to allow it to cripple us. One of the most practical lists of steps comes from the author of *How to Survive Change You Didn't Ask For*.

1. Focus on the solution, not the problem.
2. Because feeling in control is so crucial, ask, "What am I free to choose right now?"
3. Make a list of five possibilities. Give yourself permission not to have an answer at this time.

4. Give yourself credit for moving forward in a difficult situation. At the end of the day, look at what you've done.

5. Create a prayer list that is very specific. Direct your complaints to God. Sometimes all we can do when faced with a challenging change is to cry out to the heavens.

6. Minister to other individuals. Get out and help someone else. Who is the spiritual leader on your block? Is it you? Other people may need you.

7. Find someone in the same situation to help and pay attention to what you suggest they do. One of the best resources is the advice you give others. Be sure to follow your own suggestions.

8. Exercise—thirty minutes of aerobic exercise a day is one of the best ways to counteract the stress of change.

9. Tell yourself, "You can do it!" Learn this phrase in another language and find online courses to learn other languages.

10. If you find yourself worrying all the time, set aside a fifteen-minute worry time.

11. If you find yourself doing things you'd rather not, be sure to do things that you love regularly.

12. Thank those who help along the way. Reinforce what others do to help you.
13. What really matters here? On a scale of 0 to 10, what will help you keep the change in proportion.
14. Hang out with happy people. Spend as much time as possible with positive individuals.
15. Focus on the positive qualities you possess so you can roll with changes.[5]

Unfortunately, there are many who will not even admit change is occurring in their life. As irrational as it seems from the outside, they won't accept what is happening to them. This leads them to not just being stuck and immobilized—they let fear become their companion.

Another common response that is unproductive is blame. When did blame ever solve anything? It's an angry reaction as well as a way to feel relieved of responsibility. It's so easy to blame the government, politicians, educators, and so on.

It's so easy to take the responsibility off oneself and bemoan others as a way to get us off the hook, saying, "There is nothing I can do . . ." But what if you flipped the statement to, "I don't like what is happening, and I can't change the decisions being made right now, but I can . . ."?

Focusing on the problem rather than the solution can lead to feeling stuck. When you focus on the problem, you reinforce the probability of repeating it. I often ask, "Did this work for you when you tried it before?" It's like saying, "If it doesn't work, why keep doing it?" Are you willing to try a new approach? What are you doing that gives you a new and positive approach to life?

For years I have used a "Loss History" in my seminars and with individuals who are struggling with loss and grief. But have you ever thought of creating a "Change History"?

Take a blank piece of paper and draw a line in the middle of the page. Label one side *Disruptive Change* and the other *Positive Change.* Look back over the past ten to fifteen years and list the changes that have occurred in your life. You may find that some of the changes started as disruptive but led to something better. You may also find more changes occurred in 2020 than in the past fifteen years (see example of a Change History below).

CHANGE HISTORY

Disruptive Change	Positive Change
2008—Broken Engagement	
	2010—Married the man of my dreams!
2012—Moved across the country giving up dream job	
2013—Husband lost job	

Have to move back home and
live with parents

2013—First child is born

2014—Second child 18 months
later

2016—Daughter is diagnosed
with cancer—confined to
home except for doctor's
appointments

2018—Miscarriage

Late 2019—Found out
pregnant; due April 2020

March 2020—COVID-19
shutdowns

Family will not be at the
hospital when the baby is born

April 2020—Healthy baby girl!

School-age children home all
day

Husband worried about losing
job

Sleepless nights with new baby

Family cannot come to see baby

Husband didn't lose job, asked
to work at home—lots of help
with the kids

Extended family gatherings
canceled:
  Easter
  4th of July
  Thanksgiving
  Christmas

> February 2021—Parents
> vaccinated—able to visit!
> April 2021—Family together
> for Easter

As you read over your own change history, take time to pray. Thank God for the good things, and work through the unwanted changes to release their hold as you move into the future. This may be an exercise you come back to several times. And encourage your children, family members, and friends to complete this also.

As you look at your Change History, consider these questions:

- Which of these changes have come from the Lord?
- How have these changes impacted your life?
- Which of these have you prayed for or through?
- As you consider your changes and what you have done in response, what has worked, and what did you do to bring about positive changes?

- What would you do differently if you faced this change again?
- What inner resources did you use from the past? What new ones did you cultivate?
- What helped you to be positive and focused?
- Who were your supporters?
- Who are the people in your life who encourage you? Write their names. How are you praying for them?
- Who are the ones you don't want to help you? Write their names. How are you praying for them?
- What qualities do you have now that you didn't have when you faced these changes?
- How can you offer to help others?
- What can you do in an ongoing way to stay strong in your beliefs and remain strong in your foundation?

"Trust in the Lord with all your heart, and do not rely on your own understanding; in all your ways know him, and he will make your paths straight." (Prov. 3:5–6)

". . . casting all your cares on him, because he cares about you." (1 Pet. 5:7).

CHAPTER 3

You Can't Hug from Six Feet Away

I look forward to spending the summer months with my grandchildren. I couldn't wait to be with them, but I knew this summer would be different. As they played outside, I would watch through the window. When they waved goodbye, my eyes would fill with tears and my heart and arms would ache with wanting to hold them.

As humans, we crave connection, and physical touch is one of our instincts. We are born needing to experience touch. Science has shown skin-to-skin contact is one of the most essential experiences after taking our first breath. That is why a child is placed on the mother's chest moments after they're born. *God wired us for touch.* Studies have proven that physical touch boosts our immune systems, improves our psychological states, and can literally save our lives.[1]

Touch is a way of conveying love, concern, and acceptance. "It's how we connect to our parents, soothe ourselves, and show affection to others. Human touch and connection are so important that infants who don't grow up in affectionate homes are likely to have more developmental and behavioral issues than others."[2]

A few years ago, could you have imagined a *touchless culture*? Impossible? Far-fetched? Not anymore. A new disorder has been created—*lockdown disorder*. Have you ever considered how many times you touched someone during the day before the restrictions were implemented?

It's not just the isolation but also the fact that any time an end seems to be in sight, something changes and contact with others is not recommended. Even as vaccinations increase, social distancing is continued as the recommendation—and this is *not* a solution. We are created for closeness; spending all our time six to nine feet apart does nothing to build relationships or diminish fear. One college student summed it up this way: "I worry that the experience of this pandemic might convince people that we can keep living just fine while physically isolated from others. There's something about the physical presence of another human being that you can't simulate. No screen will ever replace the feeling of an arm around your shoulders. My fear going forward [is that], some of us will never come out of self-quarantine; that dread and the uncertainty will cause us to lose part of our physical connection to the world."[3]

Why is touch so important? One reason is your skin is the largest organ in your body and has two receptors. The first helps you locate, identify, and manipulate emotions. The second helps you connect with other people through emotions. It's the latter that is significant. Another reason is your mind, body, and brain are not separate from one another—they are all interrelated. When you're touched, biological changes actually occur in your brain. "Stress hormones and brain cell survival are benefited as well."[4] Touching expresses reassurance and affection. If you want to live long, you need touch.

So, how do we navigate through lockdowns, self-distancing, and life being radically changed? Even as restrictions lift, the lack of spending time with others has taken its toll. The need for touch does not change, and the choice to be touched or not is different than having the choice taken away.

The top love languages are words of affirmation and physical touch. The need for touch seems even higher during this current climate, and many are craving touch more than they normally do. Family gatherings, once a place for an affectionate embrace, have been discouraged. A warm handshake has become a fist or elbow bump, a nod or a bow. Companies sent their employees home to work, and the casual touch on someone's shoulder to get their attention or ask a question has now turned into a text or an email. As technology advances, the necessity to be physically together has decreased. But seeing someone on the computer screen is far different than sitting next to them. It feels empty. Being touched and touching someone else are the most fundamental modes of human interaction.

Touch is the most elementary tool we have to calm ourselves down. We can become *touch-starved* without it, going through life feeling restricted. Perhaps you've seen or experienced this. An example is holding back tears. Your entire body can become physically restricted when emotions are bottled up inside. A touch can free us up. One woman described her experience: "I went to a massage therapist to resolve the physical pain in my back. As she worked to get the kinks out of my shoulders, she also listened as I told her about the death of my mother. I had struggled with the loss. Although I loved her very much, I was angry with her for not taking better care of herself. As I told the therapist my story, her touch was lubrication for my soul. I was able to cry for the first time and let go as I worked through my complicated loss."[5] *Touch can open the gates of grief.*

Touch is also a way of communication. I went to my physical therapist once a week for more than two years. He must have touched me twenty times each visit. I can't imagine the results without being able to connect with physical contact. Some people even wait in their physicians' offices for a physical examination for ailments that have no organic cause. Why? They want to be touched and wait for the doctor to find the cause of the pain to make them better. Unfortunately, many of our doctor's appointments are now virtual, and touch has now become a thing of the past.

Touching enhances the nervous system of those who suffer from various illnesses as well as the immense system of those who care for them. An example is found in therapeutic back massage of those who have cancer. Touch has also shown positive results in those who struggle with any illness.[6] Touch benefits everyone from the depressed, aggressive adolescent to the elderly who are agitated and calmed by a hand massage.

Touch is one of the best ways of connecting with others and producing changes in your brain. As mentioned earlier, when we're touched, we release oxytocin, a hormone responsible for regulating positive moods and making us feel happy. It is important to find ways to cope with touch deprivation. The good news is there are ways of doing this even if the touch is not from another person. This may not be a permanent solution, but we can find comfort during this challenging time.

- Brush your hair or have a family member brush your hair.
- Massage your hands and feet.
- Massage body oil or lotion into your skin after a shower.

- Use a body pillow—the body pillow mimics a hug or cuddling with another person as well as reducing stress.
- Use a weighted blanket—a weighted blanket gives you a sense of security and helps with trauma, loss, and anxiety. It has been described as a gentle hug.
- Dance—dancing is a way to release feel-good chemicals, even if you're dancing around the house alone to your favorite song.[7]

Another way to connect, that should not be overlooked, is spending quality time with animals. Often pets are the ideal soothing mechanism. Animal sales and adoptions soared during the pandemic. Americans throughout the country have tried to fill the void of being home with a canine companion or a cuddly cat. Whether trying to fill the void of loneliness with no way to socialize, or a way to entertain children while working from home, the demand for dogs and puppies has increased.[8]

When I'm out walking my golden retriever, many times someone will come up to me and ask, "May I pet her?" That's our first inclination—to run our hands through the fur of a gentle dog. Most people don't realize the health benefits they receive from petting dogs. It has a calming effect; it lowers our blood pressure and our heart rates, and calms us down if we're stressed.

Several years ago, I was on the East Coast promoting my book, *A Friend Like No Other: How Dogs Enrich Our Lives.* This was the first of four books I've written on the joy of having a dog in your life. I didn't take my dog, but the publisher arranged for what I called a *rent-a-dog.* The golden retriever came equipped with a trainer, and as we walked through the convention hall, we ran into Joni Erickson Tada, who is a quadriplegic and has a wonderful ministry. We wanted to talk, but she had an appointment and asked us to follow her. When we arrived, the first thing she did was undo her arm from its position on her chair and place it on the head and back of the dog. The delight on her face was a gift. I'm not sure how much she could feel, but she still wanted to touch and connect with the dog.

Recently a friend shared the story of an elderly woman living in a nursing home for many years. One day he went to visit and brought his large dog. As they entered the room, the woman in bed sat up. She gestured for the dog to come closer. With a wag of his tail the dog came next to the woman. She leaned over and began to pet him. This continued for an hour, and slowly she relaxed. She told the dog the story of her life. This one-way conversation went on for some time. Eventually, she laid back down on her bed. She was surprised to see the entire nursing staff in the hall listening to her story. She asked, "Oh, did I do something wrong?"

One nurse smiled and said, "No, this was good."

As my friend was leaving, the head nurse stopped him and said, "She's been here for five years and has hardly said a word. Today she shared her story. I guess what it took was someone who listened and responded to her touch in a caring way."

I have been the recipient of the support and use of a therapy dog. Several years ago, my mother was staying in a skilled nursing facility. I visited her daily. I took my calm, loving golden retriever Sheffield with me. She would pet the dog for a few minutes and then turn to talk to me. I noticed each day there were more and more people in the lobby awaiting my arrival, looking for my dog—not me. After a time, I took Sheffield out to the lobby and said, "I'd like to spend time with my mom, but I need someone to watch Sheffield, is there anyone who could help me?" Everyone in the room lifted their hand. They all wanted to spend time with him. He was loving and gentle and would lift his paw to touch them gently and sit quietly to let them pet him.

There is one touch that most dogs want more than any other, and that is a touch from his master. My golden I have now pursues me in the evening for those touches and moans in delight as I comply. She never seems to get enough of my attention.

You and I are the same as our dogs. We long for touch. It may be from a parent, a spouse, a child, a friend, or God Himself. We can't exist without being touched. One of the worst traumas of life is that of neglect. And it did not start with this pandemic. It happens all over the world. It happens in orphanages in third-world countries where babies lie in their cribs for twenty-three hours a day starving for love and interaction.

In the New Testament, there are numerous stories of Jesus touching people and being touched. Many times, our Savior offered an embrace when a simple nod or handshake would have been enough. The Gospels are full of stories about people who sought to touch Jesus: little children, a woman suffering from hemorrhages who desperately grasped the hem of His garment, a prostitute who anointed Jesus' feet with her tears and wiped them with her hair, and even the disciple Thomas, who because of his doubt said he wouldn't believe unless he could feel Jesus' wounds with his own hands. In those days, there were many who were considered untouchable because of diseases and being ceremonially unclean. Jewish law at that time was clear. We think now how terrible that was, and yet, for safety, we now live in a culture that says, "Don't touch; you may pass on COVID." In his book *Love Beyond Reason,* John Ortberg reminds us of our Master's touch:

> The leper made no attempt to touch Jesus. The leper understood the situation. He knew the law.
>
> But notice what Jesus did: "Moved with pity, Jesus stretched out his hand and touched him, and said to him, 'I do choose. Be made clean!'"
>
> . . . Jesus did not need to touch the leper to cleanse him. He performed other miracles at a

distance; all he had to do was "say the word." The word healed his body, but the touch healed his soul. But Jesus wanted something understood.

The miracle of the touch is that Jesus was willing to share another person's suffering in order to bring about healing. This is a foreshadowing of the cross: Jesus taking on our sin so that we could take on his life. By his stripes we are healed.

In a contagious world, we learn to keep our distance. If we get too close to those who are suffering, we might get infected by their pain. It may not be convenient or comfortable. But only when you get close enough to catch their hurt will they be close enough to catch your love.

Jesus did not call his followers to live in quarantine.[9]

Though it may not be a physical embrace, Jesus still touches us today.

How do we as followers of Jesus reach out and touch those around us who are missing it so much? What we took for granted a short time ago has been taken from us. But God says, *please touch*. Touch brings healing to those who are broken. It is time for you to put your arm around a friend or embrace a child in a new way.[10] Here are some ways for you to be the one who *hugs* someone else:

Take the time to write a letter to a friend and mail it. Finding something unexpected in the mailbox will brighten their day and be a physical reminder of your care.

Take advantage of the vast variety of children's books and send a book to a child who is lonely and missing their friends.

Pick flowers from your garden or buy a small bouquet and drop them on a neighbor's porch.

Mail or email a gift card to local restaurant to a friend or family member in place of making a meal.

Use video messaging as much as possible to stay connected and make eye contact with loved ones.

Find ways to be creative and you will find yourself as blessed as the people you are blessing.

RECOMMENDED RESOURCE

Charlotte Hilton Anderson, "The Benefits of Cuddling," *Reader's Digest*, April 2020, 53; https://www.pressreader.com/usa/readers-digest/20210420/282153589101897.

CHAPTER 4

Anxiety and Worry Are Not Your Friends

Uncertainty . . . Dread . . . Fear . . . Isolation. The emotions that come with anxiety and worry are familiar to everyone and are mixed into every aspect of our lives.

"I don't know what to believe. All of a sudden, it feels like my husband is a soldier fighting daily on the front lines. He is an ER nurse in a large hospital near our home. My anxiety soared when COVID-19 patients began flooding the emergency room. The husband of my closest friend was furloughed immediately after the pandemic began, and part of me is jealous. We are thankful and blessed that he still has his job, but we're uneasy each night when he comes home. Did he contract COVID today? Will he pass it on to me or our two children? Should he hug us, be in the same room with us, or completely isolate himself? We need his paycheck but need him to be part of our family even more. There seems to be no end in sight—when will this be over? My mind is *on* constantly."

How has anxiety affected you at this time? Do you relate to any part of this story?

Anxiety has many faces—tension, nervousness, or butterflies in your stomach. Your heart could race, or it could have a positive side that alerts you and puts you on guard when you're in danger. The right amount of positive anxiety can improve memory and concentration for a short time—you may find yourself more productive with a deadline coming. But too much can leave you frozen and not able to move forward. Ancient Greeks described anxiety as opposing forces at work to tear a person apart. It can dominate your life.[1]

We live in the age of anxiety. It dominates our thoughts, influences our emotions, and drains our physical resources. It's an unwelcome guest and a disruptive intruder. Anxiety spares no one, but it has its place and purpose.

We've always struggled with this, but now even more. The world today is overshadowed by deep-rooted anxiety that feeds our fears and worries. We live in an uncertainty overload.

Anxiety is a painful uneasiness of the mind tied to an impending event. We've spent months looking outside to see if everything was still there, wondering, *What will we lose next? How will we get through this?* Daily we watched the numbers rise, wishing it weren't true. This threat caused anxiety, and at times we doubted our ability to handle it.

Whether anxiety is triggered by stress or worry—or a mixture of both—it activates the body's emergency-response system. It's a response full of fear that includes sweating, muscle tensing, rapid pulse rate, and fast breathing. We experience anxiety in both our minds and our bodies. Anxiety's close cousin, worry, resides in our minds.

Our stability has diminished. We live with the questions, "What's next?" "What can I depend on?" We wonder where the security we once had has gone. We've learned to live with "What if . . . ?" and our brains respond with more negative thoughts than positive.

> *What if* I get COVID and don't recover?
>
> *What if* I lose my job and can't afford to keep my home?
>
> *What if* my child falls behind in school and doesn't graduate?

We live in turmoil. Anxiety and worry are *joy robbers* interfering with our lives.

Habakkuk the prophet explains some common effects of worry and anxiety: "I heard, and I trembled within, my lips quivered at the sound. Rottenness entered my bones; I trembled where I stood" (Hab. 3:16).[2]

Anxiety is toxic, and worry is thinking turned into poisoned thoughts. A small trickle of fear that meanders through the mind until it cuts a channel into which all other thoughts are drained.[3] This is a misuse of thoughts that we allow to spin out of control. Where our thoughts start and end can be miles apart due to runaway thinking.[4]

Excessive worry can cause suffering, and even hinder our lives. It's as though the worry portion of our brain has a spasm and can't let go of the perceived problem to see the other side and good news is rejected.[5]

There are several verses in the Bible that speak to worry and anxiety. Luke 21:14–15 says, "Make up your mind not to worry beforehand how you will defend yourselves. For I will give you words and wisdom that none of your adversaries will be able to resist or contradict" (NIV). How will you do this?

Luke gives a command, implying that we have the capability of following it. "Make up your mind" means we have a choice as to whether *we choose* to worry or *choose not to worry*. "Make up your mind" is translated from a Greek word that means "to premeditate."

First Peter 5:7 says, "casting all your cares on him, because he cares about you." *Cast* means "to give up" or "to unload," and the cares you are casting on him are your anxieties and worries.

Isaiah rejoiced to the Lord, "You will keep the mind that is dependent on you in perfect peace, for it is trusting in you" (Isa. 26:3).

Whatever you choose to think about will either produce or dismiss feelings of anxiety and worry. Those who suffer from worry are choosing to center their minds on negative thoughts in this way. God has made the provision, but *you must take the action*. Freedom from worry and anxiety is available, but you must take hold of it. Center your thoughts on God, not on worry.

COVID-19 is a new disease, but worry is an old one—a disease of the imagination. It's a virus that slowly and subtly takes over and dominates your life. When this happens, your ability to live life the way you want is diminished. You may wonder if there are ways to change your pattern of worry and anxiety. The answer is *yes*. In Matthew 6:27 Jesus asks, "Can any of you add one moment to his life span by worrying?" The answer is *no*—remember worry is a *joy robber*. What can you do to find joy even when there is so much to worry about?

First, take control of your thought life by reading as much as you can. Two helpful resources are *Overcoming Fear and Worry*, by H. Norman Wright, and *Freeing Yourself from Anxiety*, by Tamar E. Chansky PhD. These resources can give you control of your life, especially your thought life and your brain. Your brain is under attack and needs to move from the defensive to the offensive (see *How to Keep Your Brain Healthy* by H. Norman Wright).

Then take a worry vacation by setting time aside each day to do things that you would do if you weren't worried or feeling anxious. To keep out worry put a *Do Not Enter* sign on a door in your home to remind you to keep the worry out!

DON'T LET YOUR FEELINGS RULE

Emotions arrive first and call the shots. This will cause you to react before you know why and emotions will control your day. We fear feelings because often they make the worst part of an experience appear before the rational mind catches up and brings stability to your life. Your brain is wired to feel before knowing. When you begin to worry, take a deep breath and let your rational side kick in.

Tell yourself, "The way I feel now is *not* how I'll feel later."

TAKE A DEEP BREATH

When we're anxious, we tend to take short rapid breaths, causing our body to react negatively. To counter this reaction, focus on slowing and calming your breathing. Inhale deeply through your nose and count to three before exhaling through your mouth, blowing the air out slowly. Repeat this several times until you feel your breathing pattern return to normal.

SET A TIME TO WORRY

If you find yourself worrying for the better part of the day, schedule a time to worry. Any time you start to worry, remind yourself that you have a time, from 6:30 to 7:00 each evening (set a time that works best for you), and spend that time reflecting on all your worries. The rest of the day, do not let the thoughts settle.

THE CONTAINER

A technique I learned more than fifty years ago is to use the *worry container*. Select a container and write "Worry Container" on the side. Whenever you begin to worry, take a piece of paper, write it out in detail, open the lid, put it inside, and close the lid. When you dwell on the same worry, remind yourself that you're not going to forget it because it's in the container. In time you will be able to take control of your worries without the container.

TELL YOURSELF TO STOP

During a class I was teaching on worry, I asked students to report on this exercise I had suggested. One student reported she began the experiment on Monday and by Friday she felt the worry pattern she had lived with for years was finally broken.

Take a blank index card and on one side write the word *STOP* in large, bold letters. On the other side write the complete text of Philippians 4:6–9. Keep the card with you at all times. Whenever you're alone and begin to worry, take the card out, hold the "stop" side in front of you, and say aloud "Stop!" Then turn the card over and read the Scripture passage aloud twice with emphasis.

Taking the card out interrupts your thought pattern of fear and worry occurring in your mind. Saying "Stop!" further breaks your automatic pattern of worry. Then reading the Word of God aloud becomes the positive substitute for worry. If you are in a group of people and begin to worry, follow the same procedure, only do it silently. Many who have tried this share that for the first time in their lives they've stopped worrying.

I have been using and suggesting the Stop-Think card and the Container exercises for more than fifty years and have seen hundreds find freedom from worry.

GET SPECIFIC WITH YOUR WORRY AND ANXIETY

You can also get specific with your worry and anxiety by facing it head-on. Ask yourself the following questions:

1. What worries me the most?
2. What am I actually afraid of? What do I fear?

3. What do I picture will happen? How much do I really believe it is likely to happen—10 percent, 30 percent, 70 percent?
4. What do I think is most likely to happen?
5. What steps can I take to make sure the worst doesn't happen?
6. Is this a temporary or permanent problem?

You take control by taking the vagueness out of your worry and making it more specific.[6]

Our emotions are no accident. They can be a warning sign for what is occurring in our lives as well as a source of passion and intensity. They help us monitor our needs, make us aware of good and evil, and provide motivation and energy. God has designed us in such a way that our emotions influence almost every aspect of our lives. They are like a sixth sense. The problem comes when we allow them to control us, rather than the other way around.

Using the techniques mentioned in this chapter may not help overnight, but through time and practice you can move forward and away from a life of worry. When you experience an overwhelming emotion ask yourself:

1. What is causing this emotion I am feeling?
2. If I weren't stuck on this, what would I be doing instead?

By taking control of our negative emotions, we can eradicate their hold on our minds.

CHAPTER 5

Don't Let Anger and Frustration Rule You

I am frustrated! COVID-19 is not my friend. My father broke his hip two weeks ago and has been in the hospital alone. I'm stuck here in Tennessee and I can't travel. I've been so frustrated, and today I got a phone call—my mom fell yesterday and broke her hip also. My stress level is higher than it's ever been. Dad has had a difficult time, but he understands why he is not able to have visitors. Mom had a stroke two years ago, and with her memory issues she may not understand why her family is not there with her. I also worry that when they get home, they will not get the care they need. I am just *so* frustrated!" Angry? Of course, he is.

Your feelings are like an ocean, and COVID-19 has created a storm. They come and they go . . . you're up and you're down. Just when you think they're gone for good they come back, overlapping with one another. Frustration sets in and can trigger anger, anxiety, and fear.

If anger has been brought about by frustration, it will have a tendency to disappear if the cause is removed. Like a child throwing a fit because he can't have a candy bar, he'll stop when he gets his way. If you're angry because a planned trip was canceled due to COVID, your frustration will diminish when you can reschedule. If you are angry because a child is not responding to your attempts at discipline, your anger will subside when he begins behaving.

Remember the energy of anger does not have to be unleashed in a manner that will hurt or destroy. It can be used in a constructive manner to *eliminate* the frustration. If the original frustration cannot be eliminated, many people learn to accept substitute goals and thereby find nearly as much and sometimes even greater satisfaction.

Reacting with anger is like pouring gasoline on a fire that is already blazing. Especially when you are reacting to someone else's anger. Proverbs 15:1 illustrates an appropriate response: "A gentle answer turns away anger, but a harsh word stirs up wrath."

This verse does not say that the person's anger will be turned away *immediately*, but in time it will happen. You may need to plan and practice your response in advance. If you wait until you are in the heat of an altercation, it will be difficult to change your old angry way of reacting. Visualizing and practicing the scriptural teaching in advance prepares you to make the proper response.

So . . . why do you become angry with your family members when they don't respond to you? Why do you get angry with the kids when they don't pick up their room, mow the lawn, or dry the dishes properly? Anger expressed by yelling at a son who does not mow the lawn carefully does not teach him how to do it correctly. Angry words directed to a sloppy daughter do not teach her how to be neat. Step-by-step instruction (even if it has been given before) can help solve the problem.

Another result of anger is that you become a carrier of a contagious disease. If you respond in anger, others around you can easily catch it. If you become angry with your spouse, don't be surprised if he or she responds in a like manner. You gave them an example to follow. Your spouse is responsible for his or her own emotional responses, but you still modeled the response.

I hear others say to me again and again, "Norm, I don't want to talk in an angry way to others, especially my family, but something just comes over me and I let it rip! There's a limit to what

I can take. I know I really love them, but sometimes I don't like them very much. I don't know what to do to change."

I usually respond with a question: "When you feel frustrated and angry with your family members, what do you focus on: how they reacted to what you said or how you would like them to react?"

They usually reply, "Oh, I keep mulling over what I didn't like and my destructive comments. I relive it again and again and beat up on myself for hurting them."

"Do you realize that by rehearsing your failures you are programming yourself to repeat them?" I ask.

They usually respond with a puzzled look. But it's true. When you spend time thinking about what you *shouldn't* have done, you reinforce it. Furthermore, spending all your time and energy mentally rehashing your failures keeps you from formulating what you really *want* to do. Redirecting your time and energy toward a solution will make a big difference in how you communicate with anyone. Focus your attention on how you want to respond, and you *will* experience change!

Let's consider several steps you can take to reduce your frustration and to curb words that you don't want to express. The first step is to find someone with whom you can share your concerns and develop an accountability relationship. Select someone who will be willing to pray with you and check up on you regularly to see how you are doing. If you are working through these steps as a couple, ask another couple to keep you accountable. We all need the support and assistance of others.

You also need to be honest and accountable to yourself and others about changes you want to make. Take a sheet of paper and answer the following questions. Then share your responses with your prayer partner.

- How do you feel about becoming frustrated? Be specific. How do you feel about getting angry? There are some people who enjoy their frustration and anger. It gives them an adrenaline rush and a feeling of power. Does this description fit you in any way?

- When you are frustrated, do you want to be in control of your response or to be spontaneous? In other words, do you want to decide what to do or just let your feelings take you where they want to go?

- If you want to stay in control, how much time and energy are you willing to spend to make this happen? For change to occur, the motivational level needs to remain both constant and high.

- When you are bothered by something that someone else does, how would you like to

> respond? What would you like to say at that
> time? Be specific.

There is a reason why God inspired men to write the Scriptures and why He preserved His words through the centuries for us: *God's guidelines for life are the best.* Regardless of what you have experienced or been taught in the past, God's plan works!

Write out each of the following verses from Proverbs on separate index cards (look up each verse in several other versions):

> There is one who speaks rashly, like a piercing sword; but the tongue of the wise brings healing. (12:18)

> A patient person shows great understanding, but a quick-tempered one promotes foolishness. (14:29)

> Patience is better than power, and controlling one's emotions, than capturing a city. (16:32)

Add to your card file other Scriptures you discover which relate to frustration and anger. Read these verses aloud morning and evening for three weeks and you will own them. Reading and hearing the Scriptures is important—put the two together and they will change you.

You will be able to change only if you plan ahead. Your intentions may be good, but once the frustration-anger sequence kicks into gear, your ability to think clearly is limited.

Identify in advance what you want to say when you begin to feel frustrated. Be specific. Write out your responses and read them aloud to yourself and to your prayer partner. In my counseling office I often have clients practice their new responses on me, and I attempt to respond as the other person. By practicing on me they are able to refine their statements, eliminate their anxiety or feelings of discomfort, and gain confidence for their new approach. Practice on your spouse or prayer partner

Begin training yourself to *delay* your verbal and behavioral responses when you recognize that you are frustrated. Proverbs repeatedly admonishes us to be *slow* to anger. You must slow down your responses if you want to change any habits of words you have cultivated over the years. When we allow frustration and anger to be expressed unhindered, they are like a runaway locomotive. You need to catch them before they gather momentum so you can switch the tracks and steer them in the right direction.[1]

One helpful way to change direction is to use a *trigger word*. Whenever you feel frustration and anger rising within you, remind yourself to slow down and gain control by saying something to yourself like "stop," "think," "control," and so on. Those are words that will help you switch gears and put your new plan into action.

One of the approaches I often suggest to defuse a frustrating situation is this: Mentally give the other person permission to be involved in the behavior that frustrates you. The permission-giving approach defuses your frustration and gives you time to implement a levelheaded plan.

I'm not suggesting that you give up and allow others to do anything they want to do. There are some behaviors that are highly detrimental and require a direct response.

Many people are skeptical when I suggest the permission-giving strategy. One person said, "Norm, the first time I heard your suggestion, I thought you were crazy. But I tried it. I discovered I was less frustrated. My posture was less rigid, and I was more relaxed as I dealt with that person."

Most people talk to themselves. You may even find yourself talking out loud or mumbling while you're having a dialogue with yourself. Think of your mind as a massive iPod and over time you've downloaded hundreds of statements that you can play at will. Unfortunately, you may believe them to be true. There is tremendous power in self-talk. If you have never read anything about it, you may be in for a surprise (for more information, see my book *A Better Way to Think*).

Your inner conversations or self-talk is where your frustrations are either tamed or inflamed. What you say to others and how you behave is determined by how you talk to yourself about their behaviors and responses. In fact, your most powerful emotions—anger, depression, guilt, worry—as well as your self-image as a person are initiated and fed by your inner conversations. Changing your inner conversation is essential to keeping your frustration from erupting into wounding words.

Here are some examples of anger-reducing self-talk.

- I won't take what is said or done personally.
- No matter what happens, I know I can learn to control my frustrations and anger. I have this capability because of the presence of Jesus in my life and His strength.
- I am going to stay calm and in control.
- I will respond to statements that usually trigger me with statements like "That's interesting," "I'll think about that," or "Could you tell me more about this situation?"
- I don't have to allow this situation to bother me.
- If I begin to get upset, I will take some deep breaths, slow down, delay my responses, and purposely speak softer.[2]

God's Word has a lot to say about how we think. If you have difficulty with negative inner conversations, I suggest that you write out the following Scriptures on index cards and begin reading them aloud to yourself every morning and evening: Isaiah 26:3; Romans 8:6–7; 2 Corinthians 10:5; Ephesians 4:24; Philippians 4:6–9; 1 Peter 1:13.

If you approach these steps thinking, *This will never work,* you have set yourself up for failure. Instead, think, *I'm taking positive steps toward resolving my frustration and anger. This will really make a difference in my relationship with others. I know my communication will improve as I take these steps of growth.*

To help you develop a positive attitude, take a minute to list the advantages of being frustrated and a list of the advantages of controlling your frustration. Compare the two lists. Which results do you want? You are more likely to achieve these results by following the steps above.

CHAPTER 6

Broken by Isolation

We were not created to be isolated from other people. One of the worst punishments or forms of torture is isolation. Sitting in an empty room with no windows, no human contact, and left to one's own thoughts, *solitary confinement* is used to punish and/or break down a person's will, their desire to live, to grow, and to find meaning in life. "Isolation can lead to adverse health consequences including depression, poor sleep quality, impaired executive function, accelerated cognitive decline, poor cardiovascular function and impaired immunity at every stage of life."[1]

Humans have not changed since the beginning of time. Eve was created because the Lord God said, "It is not good for man to be alone" (Gen. 2:18).

Loneliness and isolation are rarely talked about, but the pandemic changed all that. Sheltering in place affected nearly every part of our lives—employment, entertainment, education, travel, and recreation were halted as we limited our contact with family, friends, and strangers. Before the onset of COVID-19 many had difficultly defining loneliness. It has a mournful and eerie sound. It's a strange world of emptiness. But not anymore—from residents living in long-term care facilities to teens who saw their adolescence interrupted—the suddenness of minimal human interaction has affected the quality of our lives.

Several years ago, I read about an eighty-four-year-old woman who said, "I'm so lonely I could die—so alone. I cannot write. My fingers and hands pain me. I see no human beings. My phone never rings . . . I hear from no one . . . never have any kind of holidays, no kind. My birthday is this month . . . isn't anyone else lonely like me? I don't know what to do." She was living in a rundown apartment and sent a letter to the *Los Angeles Times* along with some stamps and a one-dollar bill hoping someone would either call or write to her. When the newspaper man called, she burst into tears.

Like the lady in the story above, loneliness has overwhelmed seniors throughout the country. Limited to technology many knew nothing about, they had to rely on others to connect them with their loved ones via FaceTime or Zoom or see them through a window. In October 2020 residents at a nursing and rehabilitation facility in Colorado organized a protest against Coronavirus restrictions. About twenty residents lined the street, some in wheelchairs, holding signs protesting their loneliness. They were able to see visitors, but had to stay six feet apart with no physical contact. They were missing a simple hug and holding the hands of their grandchildren.[2]

Loneliness was already beginning to take over even before the pandemic—the culprit? *Personal technology*. In 2016 one writer said:

> We live in a time when minimal interaction is the norm. We have become dependent upon devices rather than building close relationships. The more we are dependent upon this the more distance we create.[3]

Technology is useful. As businesses sent employees home to work and classes all over the country were taught online, technology was essential. We used it to keep in touch with family members during the quarantine. It became the way to see the faces of friends and family who were also stuck in their homes. But how do we keep technology from replacing in-person togetherness as we reemerge?

Some have found safety in technology because we can stay a bit anonymous. As one said, "Apps and all the other tech devices are fun. But the ability to stay anonymous on these apps makes our interactions flimsier."[4] We use emojis in our texts instead of expressing what we're feeling in words. But how often are text messages misunderstood or feelings hurt when a message is misinterpreted? Social media platforms such as Facebook, TikTok, Pinterest, and Instagram do not replace personal interaction either. Seeing what other people are doing can create feelings of inadequacy and plunge us into self-inflicted loneliness.

The problem is not the technology but our use or misuse. Computers and smart phones have become our lifeline, for good and bad. We have developed a technology mindset. Even after we put our phone down it continues to influence our lives. Interacting with our devices is not helpful for creating closeness with others. Our face-to-face dealings become stunted, as we turn to our devices for entertainment. Our opportunities for closeness are diminished. How do we find a balance in the ever-growing world of technology?

As you look back over the months of isolation, did you build closer relationships with family members or did the time together cause distance between you? And what about those outside your home—were you able to keep relationships intact. Take a moment to answer these questions:

- Whom are you close to?
- Whom are you no longer close to because of isolation?

- Are you closer to anyone now because of the pandemic?
- Did you use technology to keep in touch with family and friends?
- Did you spend more time on your phone playing games, downloading apps, or surfing the web? Did this do anything to keep you connected with others?

When you're feeling isolated and lonely, do you continue to turn to technology and devices, or do you reach out to a person? How about putting your phone away and going for a walk with a friend or meeting for coffee? Communicating with them face-to-face and sharing how you are *really* doing.

How can we overcome our loneliness as we emerge from isolation and reconnect with loved ones and create close new relationships? It's time to try something new and have meaningful conversations. The author of *Stop Being Lonely* made the following suggestions:

- Have deeper conversations—share three descriptive words that describe you and ask that they do the same.
- Distinguish needs and values from wants—has this changed since the pandemic began?

- Ask questions that foster closeness—ask questions that you would like to be asked.
- Find unifying commonalities while accepting differences.
- Talk productively about the past and the future—how has your life changed and what do you hope to accomplish in the future?
- Comfortably disclose your inner world— pick one area of your life you rarely talk about and open up unashamedly

Ways to show you care:

- Feel and identify positive and negative emotions—talk about them and work through them together.
- Experience empathy—listen and put yourself in their shoes.
- Bond deeply with another without losing your identity.
- Show someone explicitly that you care— pray for them and ask questions when you get together again.
- Handle disagreements while still communicating caring.

- Maintain the bond of caring over a long period of time.[5]

Have you tried any of these before? What was the result? Select a good friend (or relative) and make it a point to have deep conversations on a regular basis.

For closeness to occur and loneliness to disappear, we need to open our lives. A book that impacted my life forty-five years ago said, "I would like to tell you who I am, but I am afraid to tell you who I am because you may not like who I am and that's all I've got."[6] Have you ever felt like this?

Whom do you feel close to? And the emphasis is on *feel*. Who knows you—your inner world? Knowing is the act of understanding another person from their own perspective.

Who knows you in this way?

What keeps you from closeness?

Perhaps a life of honesty and disclosure begins, not in our relationships with people, but in our relationship with God. We begin by sharing with God our personal struggles, our loneliness, doubts, and fears. In Psalm 139:1–2 David says, "LORD, you have searched me and known me. You know when I sit down and when I stand up; you understand my thoughts from faraway." Read the full chapter—He is the All-Knowing, Ever-Present God. He knows you and desires a personal relationship with you. Don't hold back as you come to Him in prayer.

As your mask is slowly removed in God's presence, you discover that He accepts and loves you. In turn, He helps us shed our masks in our relationships with people. We begin to discover ourselves and attempt to understand the ups and downs of our life. And it is through the extended hands of Christ that this is possible.

How do we draw closer to God?

- Spend time in prayer each day. Be consistent and use this time to talk with God as a friend. Quiet your heart and listen. Allow Him to speak to your loneliness.
- Spend time reading the Bible each day.
- Listen to uplifting music. Begin the day with praise music—while you shower and get ready for the day.
- Join an online Bible study. One option is onlinestudy.lifeway.com/. You can study God's Word with others around the world anywhere, anytime. You can fit this into your schedule and connect with others as you study God's Word.
- Go to church and fellowship with others. Do what is comfortable for you. Whether it is indoors or outdoors, with or without your mask.

How can we combat loneliness and isolation when our world is restricted? The following are suggestions to help you cope with loneliness when restrictions are in place:

- Reach out and connect with someone. Schedule a time to talk on the phone or through video messaging. Set up a Zoom meeting to play a game or share a meal together even if it is remotely.

- Focus on what you're grateful for. Take time each day to thank God for three things you are thankful for.

- Enjoy the simple things—your morning cup of coffee, the sunshine, or the rain.

- Have your children make cards for someone who is alone or send them to a nursing home. You can also send to Operation Gratitude (operationgratitude.com), which sends them to military personnel throughout the world. A note or drawing from a child will cheer up a lonely person.

- All ages are feeling the effects of isolation. Reach out and do something kind for someone who is struggling. Not only will the recipient be blessed, but you will be also.[7]

How beautiful, how grand and liberating this experience is, when people learn to help each other. It is impossible to overemphasize the immense need humans have to be really listened to, to be taken seriously, to be understood. "Listen to all the conversations of our world, between nations as well as those between couples. They are for the most part dialogues of the deaf."[8]

CHAPTER 7

The Forgotten Grievers— Children and Teens

CHILDREN

Just imagine you're eight years old—Little League has just started and your three best friends are on your team. Your mom is visiting your grandparents because your grandma is ill, but she will be home tomorrow in time for your first game. On Friday morning you go to school and your teacher tells you school is closing because of an illness called Coronavirus. When you get home your dad tells you baseball season is postponed, and Mom can't come home for two weeks because she has to quarantine.

Now Dad is working from home, but he is always on the phone, you have nothing to do, and while you're watching TV, you keep hearing that Coronavirus is causing numerous deaths throughout the world. Mom's gone and Dad is busy. You're sad, mad, scared, and lonely, and there is no one to talk to.

Children are the forgotten grievers in our country, and death is not the only loss they experience. School closures, playing with friends abruptly coming to a halt, parental stress due to the loss of a job or loss of a family member due to Coronavirus—are some of the unexpected and sudden losses children faced from the beginning of the COVID-19 pandemic.

Loss is a natural and inevitable part of life. A key element in a child's emotional development is learning to deal with the feelings associated with loss and growing through the experience. Parents who guide their children through the troubled waters of change and grieving will equip them to handle the losses of their adult lives better. Whether the loss is a death or circumstances beyond their control such as school closures or shelter-in-place orders, children need to learn how to grieve (a resource to help you and your family is *Experiencing Grief*).[1] It is important to acknowledge their losses.

GRIEVING OCCURS IN CHILDREN OF ALL AGES

Grieving is not just for adults or adolescents. Young children show their feelings in a number of ways. Because they don't understand the significance of the loss, they may ask seemingly useless questions again and again. They may ask, "Why can't I play with Justin anymore?" "Why do we have to wear these masks? They're too hot." Concepts take time, and the concepts of unexpected change and loss haven't been fully formed yet in the children's minds. They may appear bewildered and regress in their behavior, becoming demanding and clingy. If what was lost is not returned, expressions of anger increase. They don't understand. Changes in home life, such as loss of a job or the death of a family member, can cause trauma. This further undermines the children's sense of security and raises their anxiety.

As they get older (starting at age three), children engage in what is known as magical thinking. They believe that their own thoughts can influence people and events. Fears also increase at this age. They become aware of threatening events around them. They realize their parents are worried and they become anxious too.

Children focus their attention on one detail of an experience and ignore everything else. Do you ever catch yourself doing this? Children have difficulty seeing the whole picture clearly. They don't comprehend the significance of loss.

If Grandpa is in the hospital and they can't visit, they may ask or think:

- *Does this mean someone else is going to get this?*
- *Grandpa had a headache and went to the hospital; Mommy says she has a headache too . . .*
- *Old people die; will Grandpa die too?*

When talking with your children, be sure to be clear. You must explain the difference between "very, very sick" and just sick. Explain that quarantining is to keep the germs away and is to help them.

As children get older, they develop the ability to understand loss and even death.

When faced with any type of loss, children may use denial as a coping mechanism. It's easier to act as if nothing happened. Afraid of becoming out of control, children may vent their feelings only when alone. They may appear insensitive, uncaring, and unaffected by the loss, which leaves you unaware of the extent of their grief. Children need to be encouraged again and again to share their feelings. Allowing children to see you grieve and talk about your feelings can help them work though their grief. Talking, drawing, and songs are just some ways to bring the issues to the surface.

The following are several unique features of a child's grief. As you read through these, where do you see yourself experiencing the same?

- Their emotions come out in the middle of everyday life and can't be predicted.
- Children put grief aside easier. One question may be about their grandfather's death, and a moment later they want to play their video game.
- They express their grief in actions. They may throw a fit or cry uncontrollably without knowing why. They're limited in their verbal expression.
- The losses they experience now may affect them throughout childhood. They may experience ongoing distress and deny the loss. Pieces of it last into adulthood and their grief may continue for many years. They need to know what is normal.

Regardless of the type of loss children experience, it's critical to communicate and share information in their language and level of understanding. The following eight steps are important in the grieving process.

1. *Help them diminish their fears.* Children may worry about getting sick, a family member getting sick, or have a fear of the unknown. By talking with your child about their fears, you can create a secure place so that they

can learn to feel safe again. Take time to check in with your child daily, asking questions and letting them ask questions.

2. *Children need to accept the loss, experience the pain, and express their sorrow.* Giving your children permission to grieve and encouraging them to talk will help them work through their loss. Like you, your child does not grieve on command. You may need to help them share their feelings and teach them how to express sadness. Be sure to be available and present when your child is ready to talk. Children need a sense of security. Eye contact as well as holding their hand or giving them a hug will provide comfort and reassurance. This is easier said than done.

3. *Children require assistance to identify and express the wide range of feelings they're experiencing.* They feel confused and overwhelmed by new emotions. They need your stability and will look to you for hope and support. Use Elmer the Elephant[2] and The Ball of Grief[3] to help them put words to what they are feeling.

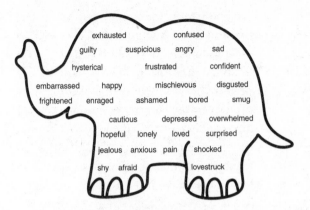

Elmer the Elephant

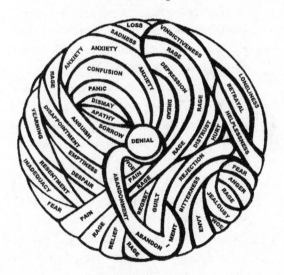

The Ball of Grief

4. *Children need to know why others are sad and why they themselves are sad.* Acknowledging these feelings lets a child know that it's *okay* to be sad. Tell them, "This is how we feel when someone dies" or "It's okay if you're upset because you can't go to school . . . or to Grandma's house." But be careful not to expect too much from your child. Allowing them to respond in their own way will help them work through their grief. They may not express their feelings in a way you would expect, but their actions may tell a different story. Help them cope by listening and working through their response.

5. *Children must be told the reason people are sad.* Without an explanation, they may think others' sadness is caused by something they did or didn't do. Start by saying, "This is a very, very sad time"; "A very sad thing has happened to Grandma"; "Mommy and Daddy are sad because . . ." If you don't talk with them, they will fill in the blanks themselves. Imagination and other children are not good resources.

6. *Encourage your child to acknowledge, remember, and review the change and losses that have occurred.* This will help them prepare for

future losses. Who taught you about loss? As an adult, were you prepared for sudden change and loss? Sheltered children don't cope as well as those who understand the ups and downs of life.

7. *Children need help in learning to relinquish and say goodbye to what they have lost.* How do you say goodbye to an entire season of football?

8. *Children respond differently to loss depending on their age and level of emotional maturity.* When they ask questions, be honest and avoid giving platitudes. Let them know it is all right to ask *why?* when bad things happen. Let them know you will get through this together. Encourage them to express their feelings with a letter or song.[4]

It is important to identify what may inhibit a child's abilities to grieve the losses he or she experiences. What have you struggled with and how has it affected your child? The following factors most often contribute to this problem (as you read this information, think of examples in your home, school, or church):

- Difficulty grieving past losses and roller coaster emotions during the ups and downs of the pandemic.

- Unable to handle and accept your child's frustration. They don't know how to respond. When your child cries do you say, "Get over it! No one had a birthday party this year."

- Your children are worried about how you're handling the changes that have occurred and attempt to protect you. Does your child comfort you, even though they're hurting?

- Children are overly concerned with maintaining control and feeling secure. They're frightened or threatened by their emotions. Do they have trouble sleeping even when they say they're *okay*? If so, read these scriptures aloud with them every night:

> "When you lie down, you will not be afraid; you will lie down, and you're sleep will be pleasant." (Prov. 3:24)

> "When I think of you as I lie on my bed, I meditate on you during the night watches because you are my helper." (Ps. 63:6–7)

> "When I am filled with cares, your comfort brings me joy." (Ps. 94:19)

> "I will both lie down and sleep in peace, for you alone, LORD, make me live in safety." (Ps. 4:8)

- The children don't have the freedom to share how they're feeling, because you are so caught up with your own struggles.
- The family fails to acknowledge and discuss the reality of loss and changes that have occurred.[5] Life goes back to normal as though nothing significant has happened.

With all that has happened, your child needs to be encouraged to take a break and do something fun. If playtime with friends is possible, it is an important type of expression for children, especially for younger children whose verbal skills are limited. Going to get ice cream, taking a walk, or going for a drive can also take their mind off the changes they can't control.

Be aware of what your children watch on television. Like the eight-year-old child in the beginning of this chapter, repeated news stories may affect your children. The terms "living room witnesses" and "CNN trauma" were coined for a reason. We spent nearly a year with the leading news story every night being the number of deaths COVID-19 caused. These stories were followed by news of riots and shootings replayed over and over again. Keeping our children informed is important, but bombarding them with the news of violence and death can cause unnecessary trauma and fear.

As adults we have a better understanding of why the shelter-in-place orders occurred. For our children this is more difficult. Be aware that your child may carry the fear that this may happen again. Be patient and continue to be available to listen and answer questions. Create habits that create closeness—reading the Bible and praying together, spending time away from the screen, planning and cooking meals as a family, etc.—they can look forward to and continue as they grow older.

RECOMMENDED RESOURCES

It's Okay to Cry, H. Norman Wright (Waterbrook, 2004)
Experiencing Grief, H. Norman Wright (Broadman & Holman, 2006)

TEENS

In May 2020 after six weeks of quarantine and online learning, one teen found herself with *extra time on her hands*. She was a competitive swimmer, a member of her high school marching band, and vice president of the class of 2023. Her social life and extra curricular activities came to an abrupt halt when her school closed and the lockdown began. Her parents saw their vibrant, athletic daughter become quiet and lonely.[6]

Our teens have been deeply affected by the pandemic. Their lives were put on hold. At the time they would naturally become more independent and begin stepping away from their parents, teens were suddenly trapped at home missing out on once-in-a-lifetime milestones and plans. Graduation, first job, moving away to college, homecoming, prom, sports, and virtually all gatherings with their peers came to a screeching halt.

The teen years are turbulent without the fear of an unknown illness and lockdowns. For some, adolescence is a time of continual crisis with few respites in between. For others, the transition is a bit smoother. But overall, adolescence is one of the most difficult transitions of life. It is a roller-coaster experience—self-doubt, feelings of inadequacy, and peer pressures are constant companions.

COVID-19 has wreaked havoc on their lives in a new way. There has been an increase in anxiety, depression, and suicide ideation. Mental health issues are on the increase. "Stress is significantly on the increase and at a level that many adults have never experienced."[7] They have been forced to give up much of their adolescence. A pediatrician and adolescent specialist suggested the following:

Listen and let them know there is no right way to act or feel right now. Anxious, sad, overwhelmed, scared, and even okay are all valid ways to feel. Give young people grace to get through these challenging circumstances without having to keep up their previous level of performance. Resist the "fix it" urge that tries to make everything better by dismissing, minimizing or replacing feelings. Help them break up the monotony with activities or make safe connections with friends to bring them joy. Show them they are not alone by sharing some of your worries and how you manage. Normalize that sometimes we need outside help and be prepared to seek help from a health-care provider and/or therapist.[8]

Adolescents need safety and security. In between childhood and adulthood their moods waffle. What they *know* is different than what they *feel*. With the major changes COVID-19 has brought to their lives, they need to know they can rely on family support—be honest with them and encourage them to share their feelings.

Teaching our teens to be resilient will not only help them cope with what they faced during the pandemic; it will help them to build life skills they can rely on in the future. The following suggestions may help:

Explain anxiety—Normalizing the "fight or flight" response can help your teen understand the surge of adrenaline and anxiety they feel when they're threatened. When your teen is feeling anxious, encourage them to focus their attention in a more productive way—going for a walk, writing, or drawing are just a few ideas.[9] Suggestions and exercises from chapter 4 on anxiety and worry can be used with teens.

Acknowledge disappointment—The list of disappointments teens faced during the pandemic is long. Allow your child to express their disappointment and acknowledge that it is okay for them to feel sad, angry, and upset that their plans and dreams were suddenly changed. Your child may need to actively grieve what was lost. Help them to take time to say goodbye in a letter, or verbally with you or a friend, to each loss they experienced. You may need to do this also. As a parent, some of your dreams for your child quickly vanished, and you may be experiencing the same sense of loss as your child.[10]

Use this time to teach your teen life skills—planning and preparing meals, how to do laundry, and budgeting and how to spend money wisely.[11]

Laughter—"Laughter truly is the best medicine, the quickest way to increase your joy and happiness levels—and is actually the antidote to stress. In a nutshell—the chemistry of stress poisons our bodies, affecting us body, soul and spirit. Laughter literally, chemically, proven scientifically, 'almost instantaneously reduces levels of stress hormones.'"[12] Be sure to laugh with, not at, your teen.

Focus on the positive—Take time each day to ask your teen to tell you something that happened that was positive as well as something they are thankful for. There may be days when this is more difficult, but work with them to look for the *good* and not focus on the negative.[13]

Encourage your teen to read the Bible and spend time building his or her relationship with God.—You may want to begin reading the Bible as a family, whether together each day or on your own. Take time to talk about what you've read. Starting a Bible study together can also instill deeper faith. Bible studies for teens and adults such as Angie Smith's *Seamless* (Lifeway, 2015) are a great way for mothers and daughters to study together.

Encourage your child to journal—They may find it easier to express themselves in writing rather than verbally. Let them keep their journaling private, only sharing when they want to.

Encourage your teen to do something new—In the beginning of this chapter, we introduced a teen who was struggling because her activities were canceled and put on hold. This wasn't the end of her story.

Her parents suggested she find a way to invest in herself and her future. While celebrating her mom's birthday with a casual picnic on the beach, she began brainstorming ideas to begin a luxury picnic business for families who wanted to celebrate as they had that afternoon. She launched her business Hoku Hospitality *as a safe way to get families to spend time together, outside of the house, doing something different and fun.*

You may see changes in your teen, and you don't want to ignore a serious problem. If you're not sure if you should step in or let them work through it on their own, consider the following signs of depression:

- Excessive amounts of fatigue even after getting sufficient amounts of sleep.
- An inability to concentrate, or becoming apathetic, falling behind on schoolwork, and unable to grasp new material.
- Angry outbursts and irritability. Your teen may not know why they're angry, but their outbursts can cause a ripple of anger throughout your home. Anger is a secondary emotion caused by fear, hurt, or frustration. When your teen is angry, instead of getting angry, ask them to identify what is causing their anger.
- Boredom or restlessness. In order to keep their mind off being depressed, they overextend themselves and keep busy. They

alternate between a high level of interest for new activities and becoming quickly disenchanted with them.

If your child is showing signs of depression and they're willing to share, listen and give empathy. Be available and supportive. If you're overwhelmed or they don't want to talk to you and their mental health is at stake, don't hesitate to connect with their pediatrician, a counselor, or church leader. Surviving and working through the changes COVID-19 has brought maybe more than they can handle on their own. Their health and safety is your first concern and as a parent you are not alone. Continue to reassure your child that you will get through this together and assure them that connecting with outside help and resources is nothing to be ashamed about.

CHAPTER 8

Building Up Others during Difficult Times

We are all in the same boat. We are not all in the same storm.

For some people it's sprinkling. This is a break. It's a breather. It's a rest. It's a pause. A time to reconnect with their families. Honestly, it's kind of peaceful.

For some it's a storm. It's a bit scary. It's disruptive. It's enough to make you stay up and watch the news and worry a bit.

For some, it's a darn hurricane. It's tearing at boards. It's pulling off roofs. It's washing them out to sea. It's dark and unknown. It's life-changing.

It's not WRONG to be enjoying a sprinkle or enduring a storm. But please don't negate the difference. Rest with your family. But don't minimize the hurricane engulfing your neighbor. Laugh when you can, but get on your knees for your friends.[1]

When the world began to shut its doors and prescribe mandatory social distancing, life changed abruptly. We were tested in every area of our lives, and relationships were strained.

Couples spending an extended period of time together—with children home, and the added stress of not knowing if they would still have a job—focused on their problems rather than finding ways to work and grow together.

In some cases, college-age children who had been on their own were forced to move back with their parents when schools closed. The stress of being under the same roof after experiencing freedom created conflict.

As the pandemic continued, we discovered that we had different views and reactions than family members and friends. For some, it was a matter of protecting themselves or family members who were more susceptible to the adverse effects of the virus. Staying at home and not interacting with others became their way of life. But others didn't see the need to isolate and continued socializing. The difference in risk tolerance created rifts in friendships and family relationships.

> How do we respond honestly and respectfully to people we disagree with?
>
> How do we adapt to difficulties and stabilize relationships that have been tested?
>
> How do we give our strength to others when they are in crisis and don't have the capability of seeing things differently?
>
> How do we let go of strained relationships that cannot be repaired?
>
> How do we respond to difficult people?

We have all encountered difficult people long before the pandemic began. You most likely know someone who fits the descriptions below:

- The critic—self-appointed complainer who is constantly chipping away at others.
- The martyr—always the victim and full of self-pity.
- The pessimist—who sees the glass half-empty.

- The steamroller—who doesn't know the meaning of the word *tact*. Their comments hurt, but they don't care.
- The gossiper—who is filled with envy.
- The taker, the workaholic, and the controller.[2]
- The relationally homeless—who is unable to find significant others to connect with or can't stay in a relationship long enough to make it work.

Does anyone come to mind?

Whenever you identify people as difficult, ask yourself these three questions:

1. To what degree must I be involved with this person?
2. To what degree do I need to be involved with this person?
3. To what degree do I want to be involved with this person?

Remember, you cannot control how another person acts, what they think, say, or do; but you can control two things—what you say to yourself about yourself and how you respond to what others say about you and do to you. Think about these questions for a minute:

1. When you think about yourself, are you hard on yourself or do you think about yourself in a fair manner?
2. How does your attitude about yourself affect how you get along with others at home, at work, or at church?
3. Who is in charge of your attitude?

Your self-talk affects your beliefs and your attitude. Have you ever caught yourself making an internal statement and then wondering where *that* came from? Some of what you say to yourself reflects your belief and attitude about yourself. But not only that; it also *creates* your attitude toward yourself. If what you say is negative or limiting, it affects how you respond to others and makes you less likely to communicate at your best or to present yourself in the best way possible. You also do not have as much energy as you need to respond in a healthy manner to others. Your energy has been used to deal with how you feel about yourself because of your internal messages.

GETTING ALONG WITH OTHERS BEGINS WITH YOU

A foundational Bible verse for all relationships is Ephesians 4:2, ". . . with all humility and gentleness, with patience, bearing with one another in love." The Amplified Bible, Classic Edition says: "Living as becomes you with complete lowliness of mind (humility) and meekness (unselfishness, gentleness, mildness), with patience, bearing with one another and making allowances because you love one another."

This verse is telling us to look past the faults of others and respond to them with humility, gentleness, and patience. This can be difficult because we tend to lean toward self-preservation when we've been wronged. We want to blame others when they hurt us. But the less we think about ourselves, the more we show love for others. How might others respond to you if you followed the guidelines in this verse when interacting with them?

The way we respond to others will affect our relationships, and one way of responding stands out more than others.

THE POWER OF ENCOURAGEMENT

The words translated "encourage" (*paramutheomai*) means to console, comfort, and cheer up.

In 1 Thessalonians 5:11 it means to stimulate another person to the ordinary duties of life: "Therefore encourage one another and build each other up as you are already doing." It suggests the idea of coming alongside a person and supporting him.

In the context of 1 Thessalonians 5:14, it seems to refer to those who are incapable of helping themselves: "And we exhort you, brothers and sisters, warn those who are idle, comfort [encourage] the discouraged, help the weak, be patient with everyone."

Hebrews 3:13 says we are to encourage one another every day. In the setting of this verse, encouragement is associated with protecting the believer from callousness: "But encourage each other daily, while it is still called *today*, so that none of you is hardened by sin's deception."

HOW CAN WE ENCOURAGE OTHERS?

To be an encourager you need to have an attitude of optimism. The *American Heritage Dictionary* gives one of the better definitions of the word *encourager*: "a tendency or disposition to expect the best possible outcome, or to dwell on the most hopeful aspect of a situation." When this is your attitude or perspective, you will be able to encourage others. Encouragement is "to inspire, to continue on a chosen course; to impart courage or confidence."

Encouragement is recognizing the other person as having worth and dignity. It means paying attention to them when they are sharing with you and not thinking about what you'll say next. It means listening in a way that lets them know they are being listened to. We listen with our eyes also.

My mentally disabled son, Matthew, did not have a vocabulary. I learned to listen to him with my eyes. I could read the message in his nonverbal signals. Because of Matthew, I learned to listen to others in the same way and came to understand what my counselees could not put into words. I learned to listen to the messages behind the message—the hurt, the ache, the frustration, the loss of hope, the fear of rejection, the feeling of betrayal, the joy, the delight, the promise of change. Listening intently encourages the speaker and allows them to trust you.

Encouragement validates what a person does or says. It lets people know they matter to you. When you encourage, you respect a person. Encouragement builds up!

Who comes to mind when you think of someone who needs encouragement? What could you say to this person? How can you surprise them by responding in a positive way they wouldn't expect?

When you are an encourager, you're looking for hidden treasure. Every person has underdeveloped resources within them. Your task is to search for these resources, discover them, and expand them. You will look at the person and care about what you discover. At first your discovery may be rough and imperfect, but your encouragement will help them develop and grow. Talent scouts and scouts for professional sports teams do this all the time. They see undeveloped raw talent, but they also see potential.

Being an encourager is not always easy. What about the difficult people we mentioned earlier? For some, their disagreeable personalities came out in stronger ways when the pandemic began. There is much to say about difficult people, but we can't cover it all. We can look at the Scriptures though, because there is a message in the New Testament encouraging us to get along with others.

Identify two people who are difficult, but still need encouragement. Describe how you will pray for them this week.

Read the following passages out loud, meditating on their guidelines:

> And let the peace of Christ, to which you were also called in one body, rule your hearts. And be thankful. (Col. 3:15)

> Finally, brothers and sisters, rejoice. Become mature, be encouraged, be of the same mind, be at peace, and the God of love and peace will be with you. (2 Cor. 13:11)

> So, the, let us pursue what promotes peace and what builds up one another. (Rom 14:19)

Sometimes no matter what you do, a person will not respond in a healthy way. The Scriptures speaks to this also. In Romans 12:18, "*If possible*, so far as it depends on you, live at peace with everyone." The New Century Version translation says, "*Do your best* to live in peace with everyone" (italics mine). It's interesting to see the qualifiers in this verse—"if possible," and "do your best." It recognizes that conflicts are sometimes unavoidable and there are people who are not willing to make peace with us. We cannot control another person's actions, but we can learn to control our response and not cause more discord. Do not respond to anger with anger, to criticism with criticism, or to discourtesy with discourtesy. There may be relationships you need to step back from, but in the process respond to them with kindness and honesty.

Being an encourager can lift others up even in the most difficult times. Your acts of kindness and building others up can affect your own outlook and impact you in an optimistic and positive way.

CHAPTER 9

Resilience: The Strength You'll Need

How do you respond to extreme setbacks?

Do you emotionally explode or become physically violent?

Do you go numb and feel helpless, becoming unable to cope with what has happened?

Do you view yourself as a victim, blaming others for the problems you're facing?

Are you flexible and able to adapt quickly to changing circumstances? Handling adversity and bouncing back to rebuild your life in a positive way?[1]

We've talked about the many challenges and changes in 2020, but how can we grow from these and cultivate resilience?

How can we face the challenges of the future with an attitude of strength and flexibility? In his book *The Resiliency Advantage,* author Al Siebert says, "Resilient survivors handle their feelings well when hit with unexpected difficulties no matter how unfair."[2] Survivors start out with the belief that they *will* be okay and things will turn out for the best. Even when their lives fall apart, they come back stronger than before.[3]

We think of survivors as being extraordinary individuals. A few are, but most are not. They are people of hope and faith, and just like you and I, they have their faults and flaws. They are like everyone else, with one exception—they have a different way of thinking. There are a number of factors that determine who survives and grows and who doesn't.

- Those who survive plan ahead in order to prepare for a loss or the unexpected. Were you able to plan for the pandemic? It hit quickly and caught most off guard not knowing what would happen next. How are you making plans for the future so you won't be surprised if another crisis hits?

- When it's not possible to plan ahead, they look at others who are resourceful people and learn from them. Who do you look to for planning for the future?

- They are not habitual complainers. They find ways to get rid of any negative feelings. How do you keep from complaining and getting rid of negative thoughts and feelings?
- They are aware of what they can do and ask for help from others when needed. Not only that, they're able to give help when others need assistance. Do you have a reliable network of people you can count on as well as being able to help others when you're needed?
- They have a desire to learn and grow. They don't want to remain where they are in life. What have you learned from 2020? How are you growing and moving forward in your life?

Our faith and relationship with God also help to determine our ability to be resilient and survive unexpected situations. In difficult times people of faith have to *believe against the grain*. In our weakness, God reveals His strength, and we can do more than we thought possible.

Sometimes when we go through difficult times, we believe God has abandoned us. He hasn't.

Sometimes when we go through difficult times, we think nothing matters. There are things that matter.

Sometimes when we go through difficult times, we think life is not worth living. It is!

Faith means clinging to God in spite of our circumstances. It means following Him when we can't see Him. It means being faithful to Him when we don't feel like it.

Resilient people say, "I believe!" and trust that:

> God's promises are true.

> God will see them through.

> Nothing can separate them from God's love.

> God has work for them to do.

Believing against the grain means having a survivalist attitude. Not only can we survive a problem, but out of it we can create something good.[4]

James 1:2–3 says, "Consider it a great joy, my brothers and sisters, whenever you experience various trials, because you know the testing of your faith produces endurance." Learning to put this into practice is a process. The passage does not say *respond this way immediately.* You need to feel the pain and grief first, before considering it a *joy.*

Another way to translate James 1:2 might be this: "Make up your mind to regard adversity as something to welcome and be glad about." You have the power to decide what your attitude will be. You can think, "It's terrible and totally upsetting—the last thing I want for my life. Why did it have to happen now? Why me?" Or you can say, "It's not what I wanted or expected, but it's here. It's going to be difficult at times, but how can I make the best of it?" Survivors don't deny the pain or hurt, but ask, "What can I learn from this? How can I grow?"

My wife, Joyce, and I learned the truth and significance of many passages from God's Word, but this passage came alive as we depended on it more and more. Our second child, Matthew, was born mentally disabled. His abilities never passed the level of a three-year-old child. He lived in our home until he was eleven and then at Salem Christian Home. At age twenty-two, Matthew developed reflux esophagitis and needed corrective surgery. Following the surgery, he developed complications and infection set in—a second surgery was needed. He developed adult respiratory disorder syndrome and did not respond to treatment. We prayed for God's will to be done. On March 15, 1990 we said goodbye to Matthew. We prayed at his bedside, thanking the Lord for our precious child and His provision of eternal life. Within an hour, the doctors came to tell us Matthew had died. God took him home that day and through the mixture of feelings, we felt at peace.

I never expected to have my only son born profoundly mentally disabled with brain damage and suddenly die at age twenty-two. But it happened.

I never expected my wife Joyce would struggle with brain tumors and die shortly after our forty-eighth anniversary. But it happened.

I never expected my daughter Sheryl would die when she was fifty-three and her husband, Bill, would die three years later. But it happened.

With each loss, I trusted the truth of Scripture. I mourned, I grieved, but through God's promises my faith endured. God has used me to minister to others through each trial I have experienced.

How can you use your trials and experiences for God's glory and to minister to others?

CHARACTERISTICS OF SURVIVORS

Survivors concentrate more on solutions and less on blame. The list of who's to blame for COVID-19 lockdowns and outcomes is lengthy. Don't play the blame game as you move into the future. Take time to look at your situation clearly and look for solutions. Make a list of possible outcomes for a variety of scenarios that could play out in your life and come up with a plan for each one. COVID hijacked the control we thought we had—being prepared for the *worst* can help us make the best out of any situation.

WHAT DOES THE FUTURE HOLD?

Situation	How I Will Handle It
The pandemic will end and life will go back to normal.	I will go back to work and make plans for the future.
Masks will continue to be required to interact with others.	I will get masks to match my outfits that are fun and make them an accessory or something to talk about.
My company will close and I will lose my job I've had for fifteen years.	Although I don't want to, I will look for a new job and maybe consider going back to school to pursue a new career.

Take time to look at what your future may look like and consider the many possibilities.

Survivors override their fears and discover new ways to make things different.

Survivors have an established pattern of enjoying life. They can laugh even during the difficult times and can take a break from the heaviness of the crisis.

Survivors adapt to change. They are *flexible, resilient,* and *adaptable.* The lack of these qualities makes a huge difference in the way a person copes with life. The more rigid the person is, the less hopeful his life is. Are you rigid or are you flexible? Ask your spouse or a trusted friend if you're unsure.

Survivors persevere. Perseverance is a mark of hope and faith. Do you persevere and keep on trying?

Survivors have healthy people in their lives who build them up and encourage them. They are also the encouragers building others up. "Therefore encourage one another and build each other up as you are already doing" (1 Thess. 5:11). Who encourages you and whom do you encourage?

Survivors recall previous times of adversity. They look at how they were able to get through it in the past and rely on their best coping strategies. How can you apply past coping strategies to the current situation?[5]

Survivors look to what they are grateful for and look for hope in their situation.[6]

Hope is not blind optimism; it's realistic optimism. A person of hope is always aware of the struggles and difficulties in life, but he lives beyond them with a sense of potential and possibility.

A person of hope doesn't just live for the possibilities of tomorrow, but sees the possibilities of today, even when it's not going well.

A person of hope can say an emphatic *no* to stagnation and an energetic *yes* to life. Hope is allowing God's Spirit to set us free and draw us forward in our lives.

There's no question that God's promises will be kept. They are certain. In Scripture, hope is solid and it is a certainty.

> "But those who trust in the LORD will renew their strength; they will soar on wings like eagles; they will run and not become weary, they will walk and not faint." (Isa. 40:31)

CHAPTER 10

Where Do We Go from Here?

We watched our atmosphere of hope turn to fear. The stability and predictability we once knew disappeared, and disruption has left its mark. We spent a year with the headlines dominated by COVID-19 cases and deaths, riots, and senseless shootings. We wonder what the future will hold—will this go away? Will we be able to go back to a version of what we used to have? We may not want to admit it, but we have become a frightened society. How do we turn our lingering fears into hope and not let them control our lives?

We were created in God's image to represent Him to people.

Like a blanket, fear covers over the image of God in us. If we hide under the cover of fear, we hide ourselves from the very things we were created to do or be.[1]

Fear internalized grows in power over us, and our sense of safety shrinks. Hope internalized gives us freedom over fear, and safety as we trust in the Lord.

If we agree with fear, it's like we are saying it's true. Fear plays movies in our head of imagined outcomes of worst-case scenarios that are not true. If we look for hope, we accept the outcome of our situation, and believe God is faithful in His promises.

The design of fear is to rob us of our courage and to stop us in our tracks, even cause us to retreat. Hope propels us forward with courage even when we want to retreat.

The enemy of our souls intends to take away our hope. That is one reason we should not give in to fear. . . .

One of the mightiest weapons in our arsenal against fear is the remembrance, remembrance of God's faithfulness. God knows that we tend to forget.[2]

Can we find hope in our new normal and not let fear take over?

Think about the choices you've made. Did you surprise yourself and learn and grow even when life was unstable? Have you learned patience? Have you learned to trust in the Lord? We may need to remind ourselves as well as let others know that there is something better coming in the future. We do not know when, but we can trust in these promises:

> "If I go away and prepare a place for you, I will come again and take you to myself, so that where I am you may be also." (John 14:3)

> "Look, he is coming with the clouds and every eye will see him." (Rev. 1:7)

Notes

Chapter 2: Perpetual White Water

1. M. J. Ryan, *How to Survive Change You Didn't Ask For: Bounce Back, Find Calm in Chaos and Reinvent Yourself* (Miami, FL: Conari Press, 2014), 10.

2. Ibid., 2–3, adapted.

3. Ibid., 200–201, adapted.

4. Megan Devine, *It's OK That You're Not OK* (Louisville, CO: Sounds True, Inc., 2017), 136–37.

5. Ryan, *How to Survive Change You Didn't Ask For*, 213–18, adapted.

Chapter 3: You Can't Hug from Six Feet Away

1. R. Mössner and K. P. Lesch, "Role of Serotonin in the Immune System and Neuroimmune Interactions" (Bethesda, MD: National Library of Medicine, 1998), https://pubmed.ncbi.nlm.nih.gov/10080856/.

2. Dr. Brian Wind, PhD, quoted in Courtney J. Higgins, *The Good Trade*, "5 Soothing Practices to Help You Cope with Touch Deprivation," https://www.thegoodtrade.com/features/managing -touch-deprivation.

3. *Westmont College Magazine*, Fall 2020.

4. John Arden, *Rewiring Your Brain: Think Your Way to a Better Life* (New York: Wiley, 2010), 210, adapted.

5. Sharon K. Farber, PhD, *Psychology Today*, "Why We All Need to Touch and Be Touched," September 11, 2013, adapted, psychologytoday.com/us/blog/the-mind-body-connection/201309/ why-we-all-need-touch-and-be-touched.

6. Arden, *Rewiring Your Brain*, 148, adapted.

7. Higgins, "5 Soothing Practices to Cope with Touch Deprivation."

8. Kim Kavin, "Dog Adoptions and Sales Soar During the Pandemic," *The Washington Post*, August 12, 2020, https:// www.washingtonpost.com/nation/2020/08/12/adoptions-dogs -coronavirus/.

9. John Ortberg, *Love Beyond Reason: Moving God's Love from Your Head to Your Heart* (Grand Rapids, MI: Zondervan, 2001), 56–58.

10. Ibid., 58, adapted.

Chapter 4: Anxiety and Worry Are Not Your Friends

1. H. Norman Wright, *A Better Way to Think: How Positive Thoughts Can Change Your Life* (Grand Rapids, MI: Baker Publishing Group, 2011), 16, adapted.

2. H. Norman Wright, *Overcoming Fear and Worry* (Peabody, MA: Rose Publishing, 2014), 8.

3. Ibid., 44, adapted.

4. Wright, *A Better Way to Think*, 219, adapted.

5. Wright, *Overcoming Fear and Worry*, 59, adapted.

6. Tamar Chansky, *Freeing Yourself from Anxiety: 4 Simple Steps to Overcome Worry and Create the Life You Want* (New York: DaCapo Lifelong Books, 2012), 77–79, adapted.

Chapter 5: Don't Let Anger and Frustration Rule You

1. H. Norman Wright, *Communication: Key to Your Marriage* (Grand Rapids, MI: Bethany House, 2012), adapted.

2. Gary Hankins and Carol Hankins, *Prescription for Anger* (New York: Warner Books, 1988), 196–98, adapted.

Chapter 6: Broken by Isolation

1. Amy Novotney, "The Risks of Social Isolation," *American Psychological Association*, May 2019, vol. 50, no. 5, https://www.apa.org/monitor/2019/05/ce-corner-isolation.

2. David Aaro, "Colorado Seniors Protest Coronavirus Restrictions: We Want to See Our Families," *Fox News*, October 14, 2020, https://www.foxnews.com/us/colorado-seniors-protest-coronavirus-restrictions-we-want-to-see-our-families, adapted.

3. Kira Asatryan, *Stop Being Lonely* (Novato, CA: New World Library, 2016), 23.

4. Ibid., 25, adapted.

5. Ibid., 4–5.

6. John Powell, *Why Am I Afraid to Tell You Who I Am?* (Grand Rapids, MI: Zondervan, 1999).

7. Katie Kerwin McCrimmon, UC Health, "Loneliness During the COVID-19 Pandemic: Fight It with Kindness," December 10, 2020, https://www.uchealth.org/today/loneliness-during-the-covid-19-pandemic-fight-it-with-kindness/, adapted.

8. Paul Tourineau, Swiss Psychiatrist, as quoted in John Powell, *Why Am I Afraid to Tell You Who I Am?*

Chapter 7: The Forgotten Grievers—Children and Teens

1. H. Norman Wright, *Experiencing Grief* (Nashville: Broadman & Holman Publishers, 2004).

2. H. Norman Wright, Elmer Elephant, *It's Okay to Cry* (Colorado Springs: Waterbrook Press, 2004), 39.

3. Wright, *Experiencing Grief*, 57.

4. Mary Ann Emswiler, MA, and James P. Emswiler, MA, MEd, *Guiding Your Child Through Grief* (New York: Bantam Books, 2000), 100–106, adapted.

5. Carol Staudacher, *Beyond Grief* (Oakland, CA: New Harbinger, 1987), 129–30, adapted.

6. Toni McAllister and Murrieta Patch, "Life Can Be a Picnic: Vista Murrieta Teen Leads the Way," January 26, 2021, adapted, https://patch.com/california/murrieta/life-can-be-picnic-vista-murrieta-teen-leads-way.

7. Rebekah Fenton, "Opinion: Covid-19 Has Wreaked Havoc on Young People's Lives—We Owe It to Them to See this Through," *The Washington Post*, January 27, 2021; https://www.washingtonpost.

com/opinions/covid-mental-health-teenagers/2021/01/27/99602ce2
-60b3-11eb-9061-07abcc1f9229_story.html.

8. Rebekah Fenton, "Opinion: Covid-19 Has Wreaked Havoc on Young People's Lives—We Owe It to Them to See This Through," *The Washington Post*, January 27, 2021, https://www.washingtonpost. com/opinions/covid-mental-health-teenagers/2021/01/27/99602ce2 -60b3-11eb-9061-07abcc1f9229_story.html.

9. Ellen S. Rome, MD, MPH, Perry B. Dinardo, MA, and Veronica E. Issac, MD, "Promoting Resiliency in Adolescents During a Pandemic: A Guide for Clinicians and Parents," *Cleveland Clinic Journal of Medicine*, October 1, 2020, adapted, https://www .ccjm.org/content/87/10/613.

10. Ibid., adapted.

11. Ibid., adapted.

12. Dr. Caroline Leaf, Cfaith, "Toxic Seriousness (Have Some Fun), adapted, https://www.cfaith.com/index.php/blog/22-articles/ christian-living/27530-toxic-seriousness.

13. Rome, Dinardo, and Issac, "Promoting Resiliency in Adolescents During a Pandemic," adapted.

Chapter 8: Building Up Others during Difficult Times

1. Facebook April 2020, author unknown.

2. Les Parrott III, *High-Maintenance Relationships: How to Handle Impossible People* (Carol Stream, IL: Tyndale, 1996), 7–8, adapted.

Chapter 9: Resilience: The Strength You'll Need

1. Al Siebert, *The Resiliency Advantage* (Oakland, CA: Berrett-Koehler Publishers, 2005), 2–5, adapted.

2. Ibid., 29.

3. Ibid., 29, adapted.

4. David W. Wiersbe, *Gone but Not Lost: Grieving the Death of a Child* (Grand Rapids, MI: Baker Books, 1992).

5. Paula A. Wallin, "On Your Mind: Coping with the Unexpected," *Penn Life, Patriot News*, posted February 19, 2013, updated January 5, 2019, adapted, pennlive.com/bodyand mind/2013/02/on_your_mind_coping_with_the_u.html?ampredir.

6. Ibid., adapted.

Chapter 10: Where Do We Go from Here?

1. John Morgan, *War on Fear: What Would You Do If You Were Not Afraid?* (Lake Mary, FL: Creation House, 2016), 62.

2. Ibid., 36.